Real Prenatal Nutrition

Essential Nutrients for a Healthy Baby and Mother

By

Dr. Stephanie L. Stewart

Table of contents

Introduction

A healthy diet is crucial during pregnancy, as is widely recognized. Most people are aware of this and wish to do what they can to support their baby's development, but there is sometimes conflicting advice on the foods that are best to eat. The best advice on maintaining a strong immune system for pregnant moms and their unborn children can be found in this amazing book on PRENATAL NUTRITION.

Chapter1

Real food is what?

Real food is food that has not been processed and has grown in soil. Think of real food as "regular" food—the kind that our great-
grandparents consumed before man discovered how to produce processed foods with artificial preservatives and colors to make a lot of money. Your great grandma would recognize real food (I think many young grandparents grew up on processed foods) by now.
In the definition of real food, nothing is considered bad; real food examples include steak, kale, beans, bread, and yogurt. Natural nutrient density makes a diet based on real food the best choice for pregnant women. It doesn't take a nutritionist to explain that a diet high in whole foods (such as fruits, vegetables, nuts, seeds, and legumes) is healthier for you than one high in processed foods (such as pasta, cereals, crackers, chips, and sweets).

Six reasons why you should eat real food during pregnancy

1. Increase Intake of Micronutrients

I approach prenatal nutrition by reverse engineering what to consume based on the micronutrient requirements and where we can find them in real food. Contrast this with conventional advice, which usually emphasizes eating a specific number of servings from each food group or depending on fortified foods to meet nutrient requirements. According to research, women who obtain most carbohydrates from whole foods with a low glycemic index (such as vegetables, nuts/seeds, berries, and legumes/beans) consume much more micronutrients. Contrarily, women who consume more starch—even in the form of "complex carbs" like whole grains—have lower intakes of vitamins and minerals, probably due to the foods they replace, which are higher in nutrients. Examples include substituting zucchini noodles for spaghetti, grains for lentils in a soup, and crackers for an apple and nut butter instead of a snack. Intake of micronutrients is also higher in women who follow an omnivorous diet or one that includes some animal products (eggs, meat, poultry, fish, dairy, etc.). This is especially true for several nutrients, such as vitamin B12, glycine, choline, and DHA, which are typically hard to come by. For instance, people who eat eggs often consume twice as much choline as people who don't.

In contrast to omnivorous women, 62% of pregnant vegetarians typically have vitamin B12 deficiencies(Note: Because it can only be found in foods derived from animals, vegan women must take a vitamin B12 supplement.).The amounts of DHA in plasma, blood cells, breast milk, and tissues are markedly lower among vegans and vegetarians compared with omnivores, according to a 2009 overview of the data on vegetarian diets and DHA status. If you don't eat seafood and don't want to take fish oil, I urge you to look for a DHA supplement derived from algae (flax, chia, and other plant sources of omega-3s do not provide DHA).

2. Prevent anemia

Pregnant women's needs for iron rise by roughly 50%, and if they cannot meet these demands, many develop anemia. Preeclampsia and premature labor are just two of the pregnancy issues for which anemia increases your risk. Additionally, it may interfere with your thyroid's operation and impair your child's brain growth. 5 One study found that babies whose mothers were anemic during pregnancy had delayed cognitive development when tested at ten weeks and nine months. Thankfully, iron can be found in plenty of whole foods. Heme and nonheme types of iron are both present in the diet. While only 2-13% of non-heme iron is absorbed, heme iron is absorbed much better (at least 25% of what is in the food is). 7 Animal meals include heme iron, but plant foods have non-heme iron. For this reason, it's a good idea to regularly consume some animal foods high in iron in your diet.

The following foods are some of the best sources of heme iron:

- Liver from chicken: 9.9 mg
- Shellfish: 5.7 mg
- Liver of beef: 5.6 mg
- Heart of beef: 5.4 mg
- Pork - 3.8 mg
- Bison meat, ground: 2.7 mg
- Salves: 2.4 mg
- Beef patty: 2.3 mg
- 2.3 milligrams of clams
- Sheep - 1.7 mg
- Turkey, ground - 1.7 mg
- Legs of chicken: 1.2 mg

You can put the list above into perspective by remembering that 27 mg of iron per day is required during pregnancy. Women who eat a vegan diet ought to think about taking an iron supplement. According to some research, Spirulina algae may help prevent anemia; thus, vegetarian or vegan ladies should also consider this.

3. Postpartum Recovery Is Faster

I'm aware that this doesn't fit with most pregnant women's dietary plans, but as a toddler's mother, I can guarantee you that once your kid is born, you'll be glad you ate healthily. Breastfeeding is extremely demanding; recuperating requires substantial nourishment, and giving birth is like a marathon. Your body tends to lose nutrients during pregnancy, so the better fed you are, the quicker your body will recover after giving birth.

Your body requires more nutrients as your uterus contracts again, your skin regains flexibility, and your joints and ligaments adapt to life after pregnancy. This comprises vitamin C (which helps collagen crosslink and so helps your skin tighten back up faster and speeds healing of perineal tears/surgical wounds), collagen/gelatin (for the amino acids glycine and proline), and iron (which replaces from blood loss). While eating them postpartum to hasten recovery is crucial, it's shrewd to incorporate them into your diet as early as possible throughout your pregnancy. Bone broth, grass-fed beef, lamb, dark meat chicken soups and stews, and foods strong in vitamin C like bell peppers, strawberries, broccoli, and kiwis are all recommended.

4. Heart well-being

Magnesium and heart-healthy fats are only two of the heart-healthy minerals and antioxidants that are abundant in real food. Congestion of blood vessels is one of the primary causes of heart disease; thus, eating a diet high in nutrient-dense, unprocessed foods may also help lower inflammation.

5. Full of fiber

Numerous health advantages of fiber include improvements in digestion, metabolism, and feelings of satiety. Along with beans and legumes, foods like avocados, chia seeds, flaxseeds, and blackberries are particularly high in beneficial fiber.

Since fiber from whole foods keeps you satiated longer and provides you with additional nutrients from fruit or vegetable, it is preferable to take a fiber supplement.

6. Aids in blood sugar control:

For a diabetic patient or someone at risk of diabetes, eating a diet rich in unprocessed animal products and fiber plants may help lower your blood sugar levels. People with diabetes or prediabetes participated in a 12-week trial in which they had a paleolithic diet consisting of fresh meat, fish, fruits, vegetables, eggs, and nuts. They saw a 26% decrease in blood sugar levels.

Chapter 2

Nutrients essential for pregnancy

As you are surely aware, pregnancy causes many physical and hormonal changes in the body. You'll need to choose healthy foods from various sources to sustain you and your developing baby. Eating a nutritious, balanced diet can make you feel better and provide you and your baby with what you need. You must consume all the nutrients you require because food is your baby's primary source of nutrition.

The positive aspect is that? These dietary recommendations are simple to follow and offer a variety of delectable foods. You can quickly create a healthy menu, even in the face of hunger.

Additional nutrients there is no surprise here: Because you are feeding a brand-new human being, your body has greater nutritional needs while pregnant. While it's not true that you should "eat for two," you still need additional vitamins and macronutrients to support you and your kid.

Vitamins and minerals are micronutrients, dietary components that are only needed in very small amounts.

Macronutrients are nutrients that offer energy in the form of calories. We are discussing fats, proteins, and carbohydrates. Following are some broad recommendations on a few significant nutrients that should be modified according to your needs:

Daily nutrient requirements for expectant mothers

- 1200 milligrams of calcium (mg)
- 600–800 micrograms of folate (mcg)
- Protein 70-100 grams (g) per day, rising each trimester, containing 27 mg of iron

The majority of pregnant women can satisfy these high nutritional requirements by selecting a diet rich in a variety of nutritious foods, such as:

- Complex carbs and proteins
- wholesome fats, such as omega-3s
- minerals and vitamins

What to eat and how much

Your aim? Consume various foods to meet your and your infant's nutritional needs. It is merely slightly more intense than a typical healthy eating regimen. In reality, it's quite fine to eat as usual during your first semester, then boost your daily calorie intake by 350 during your second trimester and 450 during your third as your child grows.

Avoid highly processed junk food as much as you can. For instance, soda and chips have no nutritional benefit. Fresh fruits, vegetables, and lean meats like chicken, fish, beans, or lentils will be better for you and your kid. This does not imply that you must abstain from all of your favorite foods when you are pregnant. Just make sure to balance them out with healthy foods to ensure you get all the vitamins and minerals you need.

Protein
The normal development of a baby's tissues and organs, especially the brain, depends on protein. Additionally, it aids in the

development of uterine and breast tissue while pregnant.

Even your blood supply is affected, making it possible to give your kid extra blood.

Every trimester of pregnancy will increase your requirement for protein. According to research, pregnant women should consume significantly more protein than what is now advised. It's time to serve more salmon teriyaki, jerk chicken, hog curries, and shrimp fajitas. Depending on your weight and your trimester, you'll need to eat between 70 and 100 g of protein daily. Find out specifically how much you require by speaking with your doctor.

Among the best sources of protein are:
- Lean pork, chicken, and beef
- Salmon \snuts
- Almond butter
- Beans with cottage cheese

Calcium

Calcium helps to support your baby bones and control how much fluid your body uses. Pregnant women need 1,000 mg of calcium daily, ideally in two doses of 500 mg. You'll probably need more calcium in addition to your standard prenatal vitamins. Milk, yogurt, cheese, low-mercury fish, and seafood like salmon, shrimp, catfish, and canned light tuna are all excellent sources of calcium.

Chapter 3

Foods that promotes a healthy baby

Being pregnant is a beautiful experience, yet, it can also present several unique physical and mental challenges. Maintaining a healthy and balanced diet is crucial to keep both the mother and the unborn child healthy during pregnancy. Your body requires more nutrition during this time to improve your baby's wellbeing. In fact, throughout the second and third trimesters, you need to consume 400 to 500 more calories daily. Your risk of having a complicated birth is increased by poor nutritional choices, which can also make you overweight. To meet the unique nutritional needs of the unborn child, pregnant women must take additional care with what they consume during this time. In other words, eating nutrient-rich and healthful foods will keep you and your unborn child healthy. Additionally, it makes weight loss after childbirth simple.

Thus a list of 10 foods you can consume while pregnant:

Dairy goods

Dairy products should be consumed in large quantities during pregnancy. It enables you to meet the increased need for proteins and calcium that supports the development of your fetus. To keep your baby healthy, drink more greek yogurt, paneer, and ghee while consuming at least one glass of milk daily.

Eggs

proteins, and minerals, eggs are often referred to as superfoods. Eggs are beneficial for the developing infant because they include proteins, which help the fetus' cells grow and repair themselves. Additionally, eggs contain a significant amount of choline, which is crucial for the unborn child's brain and nervous system development. The nutrients folic acid, calcium, potassium, and vitamin B6 are all abundant in bananas. They also aid in increasing energy because they are high in antioxidants. They can thus be a healthy addition to your diet during pregnancy.

The sweet potato

Beta-carotene, which is turned inside the body into vitamin A and is necessary for forming cells and tissues, is found in sweet potatoes in high concentrations. Additionally, vitamin A enhances vision and builds immunity. Therefore, increasing sweet potato consumption can benefit the mother and the unborn child.

Legumes

Lentils, soybeans, peas, beans, chickpeas, and peanuts are all considered part of the legume family of foods. They are a great source of iron, calcium, folate, plant-based fiber,
protein, and other essential nutrients for pregnant women. Your kid will be healthy at birth and will be protected from numerous diseases and infections in the future if you get enough folate.

Nuts

Nuts are an excellent choice for a pregnancy snack because they are tasty and packed with healthy fats. They provide proteins, fiber, and other vital nutrients necessary for the baby's development and brain-boosting omega-3 fatty acids.

Citrus juice

Of course, you can fill up on orange juice's folate, potassium, and vitamin C. It can give your child the nutrition they need, preventing different birth abnormalities. Orange juice's vitamin C concentration will improve your baby's body's capacity to absorb iron as a result, including one glass of orange juice in your daily meal.

Leafy vegetables

Leafy vegetables are nutrient-rich and, as we all know, can aid the body ward off many ailments. Leafy vegetables are a fantastic addition to your pregnancy diet since they are a great source of antioxidants, calcium, protein, fiber, folate, vitamins, and potassium.

Oatmeal

Numerous health advantages of oatmeal exist. All of us, notably pregnant women, need to consume carbs because they can give us quick energy to carry out everyday tasks. A good supply of carbohydrates, selenium, vitamin B, phosphorus, and calcium is oatmeal. So while you're pregnant, eat it for breakfast.

Salmon

Omega-3 fatty acids are abundant in salmon and are excellent for heart health. For women who are expecting, getting adequate omega-3 in their diet is crucial since it aids the fetus's brain and vision development. Vitamin D, which is crucial for immunity and bone health, is also abundant in salmon.

Which foods should you avoid while expecting?

Not all foods are suitable for consumption while pregnant. Some foods may be harmful to you or your child due to how they were prepared, the bacteria or chemicals they contain, or all three.

In moderation, the following foods are not safe to consume during pregnancy:

Tiny quantities of mercury in fish:A metal that can harm your unborn child is mercury. Fish absorb mercury from the water they swim in and from the fish they eat, which contain mercury. You can give the metal to your unborn child while pregnant if you consume fish that contains mercury. This could harm your baby's brain and impair their ability to hear and see. Eat a moderate variety of low-mercury seafood per week when pregnant, such as shrimp, salmon, pollock, catfish, and canned light tuna.

Additionally, 6 ounces of albacore (white) tuna per week are acceptable. If you plan to eat fish, cook until the internal temperature reaches 145 degrees and check if it flakes. Scallops, shrimp, and lobster should be milky white. Cooking should continue until the oyster, mussel, or clam shells open.

Caffeinated foods and beverages.

Your daily caffeine intake should not exceed 200 mg. This roughly equates to one 12-ounce cup of coffee or 112 8-ounce cups. Even though you conceive coffee cups as the same size, they are not all the same size. When purchasing a cup of coffee or tea, especially, check to see how many ounces it contains. Try drinking decaffeinated coffee instead of ordinary coffee, which contains only a minimal quantity of caffeine. Tea, energy drinks, chocolate, soda, and several over-the-counter medications all contain caffeine. To find out how much caffeine you're consuming, read the foods, beverages, and medications labels.

What foods must be avoided at all costs while pregnant?

Avoid consuming these items while pregnant. They could seriously injure you and your unborn child!

Some types of fish and meat

Meat that is raw or underdone, such as beef, poultry, and pork. This includes hotdogs and deli meat (like ham or bologna). If you eat hotdogs or deli meat, ensure they are piping hot, or stay away from them altogether, specifically shellfish and raw fish, and eat sushi only if the fish has been grilled. Also, stay away from raw oysters, sushi, and ceviche. Before consuming any fish you have caught, always check with your local health authority. Smoked fish, meat spreads, or chilled pates is alright if prepared into a dish like a casserole. Also acceptable are pates that are shelf-stable and can be kept without refrigeration.

Unpasteurized milk, juice, and any food products prepared with them

Store-bought salads like chicken, egg, or tuna salads, unpasteurized soft cheeses like brie, feta, camembert, Roquefort, queso Blanco, and panela

Herbal medicines and beverages, such as teas:

Herbs, which are plants used in cooking or medicine, are utilized to make herbal goods. Herbal products are not well understood enough for us to determine whether using them while pregnant is safe. It is therefore advised to avoid using them when pregnant.

Clay, starch, paraffin, and coffee grounds are non-food substances. Tell your doctor if you have a craving like this for something other than food.

Alcohol: There is no established safe level of alcohol consumption during pregnancy.

Chapter 4

Maintaining a healthy immune system

Expecting mothers are more prone to illness and infection. So pregnant women have to deal with a compromised immune system due to the body's attempt to safeguard the unborn child. Fortunately, you may strengthen your immune system without endangering the unborn child by eating a few nutritious foods, exercising regularly, and taking supplements. Zinc and vitamin D are two excellent vitamins to aid your immune system while you're pregnant. Beyond food and supplements, getting a good night's sleep, engaging in regular exercise, and lowering stress levels are some of the greatest strategies to boost your immune system. Your attitude greatly affects your health and your unborn child's health.

What are supplements and vitamins?

Your body needs several different vitamins. Vitamins are organic substances your body can't produce on its own yet are required in very small amounts. Most of the vitamins you require come from food, except vitamin D, which your skin produces from sunlight. Dietary supplements are complementary treatments that may provide nutrients that are lacking in your diet. Multivitamins, individual minerals, fish oil capsules, and herbal supplements are a few examples.

Vitamins and minerals

Prenatal nutrition is essential for your baby's healthy growth and development. It would be best if you ate enough nourishment to suit your and your infant's demands. You require more protein, folate, iodine, iron, and certain vitamins when pregnant. For instance, folate(also known as folic acid as a supplement) helps prevent neural tube disorders, such as spina bifida.

Iodine is necessary for the growth of the neurological system and the brain. Iron aids in the prevention of both low birth weight in the infant and anemia in the mother. Additionally, crucial nutrients are vitamin B12 and vitamin D, which assist the growth of the baby's skeleton and neurological system, respectively (D). Adequate vitamin C intake also aids in better iron absorption from food.

Should I be taking a supplement?
Taking folic acids, iodine, and vitamin D supplements is advisable.

The other nutrients you require should be available to you if you eat a healthy diet, which is vital. But in addition to folic acid, iodine, and vitamin D supplements, certain expectant mothers could also require other nutrients. Your physician might suggest taking a supplement if you have a deficiency.

For instance:
Vegetarians and vegans who don't obtain enough vitamin B12 might consider switching;

- If you don't consume enough calcium from dairy products or other calcium-rich meals, which is essential for bone health,
- If your iron levels are low
- If you might be deficient in omega-3 fatty acids, for example, if you don't eat much seafood

Consult your doctor if you're unsure whether you need a supplement.

Supplements during pregnancy

A multivitamin is a blend of various vitamins and minerals often swallowed as a pill. Certain multivitamins are created specifically for expectant mothers (prenatal multivitamins). However, they do not serve as a replacement for a balanced diet. Even if you take prenatal multivitamins, consuming a balanced diet is still crucial. Avoid consuming non-pregnancy-specific multivitamins when pregnant.

Watch out for certain vitamins.

Each vitamin is only slightly necessary for your body, and larger amounts are not always preferable. In reality, overindulging has negative effects. For instance, taking excessive amounts of vitamins A, C, or E can be harmful. Pregnancy is not the time to take these vitamins as supplements. Additionally, it's advised to avoid foods like liver and liver-derived products like pâté that may be extremely high in vitamin A. It's best to see your doctor before taking any supplements, just as you should before taking any medications while pregnant. Research has confirmed that probiotics may help manage blood sugar levels during pregnancy and that taking omega-3 supplements may help lower the chance of early birth. But it's unclear whether using these supplements has more advantages than disadvantages. It is recommended to avoid them unless your doctor has prescribed them up to now, especially during the first trimester of pregnancy. Because they are considered "complementary medicines," dietary supplements are not subject to the same scrutiny or regulation as other medications.

Chapter 5

Exercising during pregnancy

The American College advises pregnant women of Obstetricians and Gynecologists (ACOG) to engage in at least 30 minutes of moderate activity each day, most (if not every) day of the week.

What is included in those thirty minutes? Three 10-minute walks spread throughout the day are just as healthy for your heart and overall health as 30 minutes on the treadmill or cycling at the gym. Even non-exercise activity counts toward your daily targets, such as 15 minutes of light yard work and 15 minutes of vacuuming. Even if it's true that now isn't the ideal time to start how to water ski or sign up for a horse-jumping competition, the majority of women can still participate in most exercise activities. If you had a basketball-sized belly, you'd struggle to perform several exercises prohibited during pregnancy (like mountain biking or downhill skiing). However, before beginning any fitness routine while pregnant, ensure you receive the go-ahead from your doctor. Exercise is not advised during pregnancy if certain problems exist, including placenta previa, incompetent cervix, ruptured membranes, and severe anemia.

Best aerobic exercises during pregnancy
If your doctor gives the go-ahead, you can think about the following cardiovascular workouts to improve blood circulation, muscle tone, and endurance (which you'll be grateful for come delivery day).

Swimming
The ideal pregnancy workout may be swimming and water aerobics. Why? You will feel lighter and more agile in the water since you weigh less there than on land.

Swimming in the pool may also aid nausea relief, sciatic pain relief, and ankle swelling. Additionally, because your baby is floating alongside you, it is easy on your joints and ligaments as they become more flexible due to pregnancy hormones in your body. Just be cautious when stepping onto slick pool decks, and slide or step into the water rather than diving. The bubbles inside the body when you abruptly shift altitudes under the water pressure are too much for your developing baby to endure, which is why scuba diving is strongly discouraged. Additionally, your center of gravity will probably be off as your pregnancy advances. As a result, diving doesn't have a positive impact that justifies the danger

Walking

Walking when pregnant is the easiest workout to fit into your hectic schedule. And you can keep working out until the day of your delivery (or even on that day if you want to speed up the contractions). Furthermore, you only need a pair of decent shoes and can participate without extra tools or a gym membership.

Running

Want to move a bit more quickly? With a doctor's approval, experienced runners can continue their routine during pregnancy. Never overdo it; stick on level ground (or a treadmill). During pregnancy, loose ligaments and joints can make running tougher on your knees and increase your risk of injury. Pregnant women should stick to ellipticals, stair climbers, treadmills, and rowing machines. Set the tension, inclination, and pace to a comfortable level for you. Be aware that you can encounter more resistance as your pregnancy goes on (or not; listen to your body). You'll need to pay more attention to where you step when using stair climbers and treadmills to prevent falls.

Group lessons in aerobics or dance
If you're a beginner, low-impact aerobics and dance workout courses like Zumba are terrific methods to raise your heart rate and release endorphins. Avoid any tasks that demand precise balance while your abdomen grows. If you're an expert athlete, pay attention to your body, stay away from jumping or other high-impact activities, and never push yourself to exhaustion while working out. Choose the water-based version of aerobics if you've never worked it out before; it's great for pregnant women.

Cycling inside

If you had been spinning for at least six months before becoming pregnant, you should be permitted to keep doing it as long as you scale back your workout and get your doctor's approval. Since you may bike at your own pace without falling or putting stress on your ankle and knee joints, indoor cycling can be a great form of exercise. Be sure to keep your teacher in the loop of your pregnancy, and skip a sprint if you start to feel too hot or worn out. To lessen the strain on your lower back, adjust the handlebars so that you sit up straighter and not lean forward. When climbing hills, sit down since it is too strenuous for expectant mothers to stand. Take a break from spinning if it becomes tiresome until the baby is born.

Tips for pregnancy safe workouts

Already a gym rat? Don't go overboard
When working out for an extended period, always exercise in a cool setting. Get warm and get cool. By ensuring that your heart and circulation aren't suddenly overworked, warming up, you lower the risk of injury. Finish with a few minutes of walking and some downtime before tackling the rest of your day because stopping abruptly causes blood to become trapped in the muscles and lowers blood flow to other parts of your body (including your baby).

Be aware of your body
Never overwork yourself while exercising when you are expecting. The secret to determining whether you are overdoing it is not to check your pulse. Rather, pay

attention to your body: Pain or tension are not good; if it feels good, it generally is alright. Sweating a little is fine, but becoming saturated is bad. While strenuous activity is acceptable for expectant mothers, keep your intensity to a maximum of 13 to 14 on a scale of 20; you should only exercise so hard that you can still speak while moving. And when you're done, you ought to feel energized rather than exhausted.

Recognize when anything is off:
Stop exercising if you get calf pain, edema, or muscle weakness that affects your balance. If you experience any unusual pain (from your hips to your head), a cramp that won't go away when you stop, regular painful contractions,

chest pain, a very rapid heartbeat, difficulty walking, a sudden headache, lightheadedness, increased swelling, bleeding, or a decrease in fetal movement after week 28, you should call your doctor right away.

Keep your back free:
After the fourth month, avoid exercises requiring you to stand motionless for extended periods or lie flat on your back. Your growing uterus' weight may compress blood arteries, limiting blood flow. Prevent particular actions. Full sit-ups and double leg lifts exert an abdominal pulling; therefore, it's usually best to avoid these. Additionally, avoid exercises that call for deep backbends, extensive joint flexion or extension, jumping, bouncing, abrupt changes in direction, or jerky actions.

Take a sip:
Drink at least an additional full glass of water for every half-hour you sweat, more in hot weather or if you're sweating heavily. Pack a snack, start drinking water ideally 30 to 45 minutes before exercising, and keep drinking water throughout and after your workouts. Enjoy a light protein-carb snack before and after workout sessions to prevent low blood sugar, which can result from high-intensity exercise or exercise lasting more than 45 minutes.

Dress comfortably:
Sports bras that support your breasts without pinching should be worn along with loose, breathable, stretchy clothing. To lower the danger of accidents or falls, don't forget to replace your sneakers if they are getting old.

Stay inspired:

It's rather easy to select a pregnancy exercise program that is effective for you: Choose an activity that you genuinely enjoy, and think about varying your routines to keep things fresh. In this manner, you'll increase your likelihood of motivating yourself to head for the yoga mat, even on days when you'd prefer to lounge on the couch.

Remember that there are many more ways to keep in shape while pregnant. Always confirm with your practitioner what is okay and what is not for you if you have any doubts about what is safe. When exercising, try not to be too hard on yourself, and don't forget to have fun!

Final thoughts:

Pregnancy is one of the nutritionally toughest times. You are encouraged to prepare a suitable diet, obtain enough vitamins, and take supplements for your health and the unborn child's wellbeing. Avoid using drugs, alcohol, or tobacco products while pregnant. I aim to provide you with additional details about REAL PRENATAL NUTRITION. Stay healthy!